Okinawa Diet Cookbook

Secret to a Long and Happy Life

Mary H. Johnson

Contents

Chapter One

Okinawa is a Japanese island in the Pacific.

The island of Okinawa is one of Japan's biggest. Churashima, or "beautiful islands," is its nickname. It's also known as one of the Blue Zones, which refers to parts of the globe where people are believed to be the healthiest due to low rates of heart disease, cancer, diabetes, and obesity, as well as the longest life expectancy.In reality, Japan boasts the world's highest life expectancy, with women living to 90 years old and men living to 84. (In the United States, it's 81 and 76, respectively.) According to the Okinawa Research Center for Longevity Science, Okinawa has the world's highest concentration of centenarians (those who are 100 years old or older) per 100,000 population (ORCLS). They've been studying centenarians for decades, so it's evident they're on to something—starting with their nutrition.The Okinawa Diet: What Is It?The most essential thing to remember is that the Okinawa diet is an eating style rather than a diet plan, similar to the Mediterranean diet.Native Okinawans eat a nutrient-dense, low-calorie diet. Okinawans don't consume a lot of meat, dairy, or wheat, yet they don't limit themselves to any specific foods. Aside from that, this diet has two distinct features. To begin with, it's mostly made up of plants. Meat is more of a condiment than a main entrée for Okinawans. So, on this diet plan, you may consume meat and fish in small amounts.Vegetables are abundant in the everyday diet, including sweet potatoes, pumpkin, bell peppers, bitter melon, and seaweed. "This diet is heavy in carotenoids, which may decrease inflammation and increase immune system functioning, and it's rounded out with tofu and mushrooms. They still consume rice, but in fewer amounts than a conventional Japanese diet, choosing yellow or purple sweet potatoes as a carb source."The 80/20 rule is the second most important aspect of the diet. (No, not the cheat meal 80/20 rule.) In Okinawa, people seek to eat until they're satisfied but not entirely full (thus the 80 percent). Think of it as eating dinner and leaving space for dessert, but then not eating the dessert.

Chapter Two

WHAT DOES IT MEAN TO LIVE IN A BLUE ZONE?

Mary H. Johnson, a National Geographic fellow, author, and adventurer, invented the phrase "Blue Zones" in 2004 to describe areas where locals live longer than the world average.Icaria in Greece, Sardinia in Italy, the Nicoya Peninsula in Costa Rica, Loma Linda in California, and Okinawa are all Blue Zone locations with similar diets.Limiting red meat intake in favor of modest amounts of fish or plant proteins, as well as not overeating and eating the majority of the day's calories in the morning and afternoon, are all considered to help people live longer.While the natural estrogens in tofu and other soy products, flax, legumes, and broccoli are considered to contribute to the lifespan of Blue Zone and Okinawan women in particular, plant foods are rich in fiber, which considerably decreases the risk of cardiovascular disease and some malignancies.A "moai" is a lifetime circle of friends that assist each other until old age. This notion stems from the ancient tradition of yuimaru, or mutual aid, which helped sustain community members in the greatest need.Loneliness has a substantial influence on physical and mental health, and studies show that tight-knit communities and frequent socializing may prevent depression in elderly people. Now, Okinawans create moai as helpful social organizations, but members continue to assist one another as much as possible.Socializing and staying are also important in the Mediterranean and other Blue Zone locations.Exercise, frequent social interaction, and good nutrition all come together to promote overall health.

Chapter Three

Okinawa Diet Health Benefits

The Okinawa diet is generally considered healthy and can be followed by anyone; it consists of eating whole, unprocessed foods with a high water content due to the fresh produce, as well as being high in fiber and carbs and low in overall calories and fat—characteristics that, despite the rise in popularity of high-fat diets like keto, may help with weight loss and maintenance (the ORCLS was formed to study the impact of diet on Okinawan centenarians).The Okinawa diet is rich in vitamins, antioxidants, and fiber, all of which have been found to reduce inflammation.The fundamental attraction of this eating pattern is the attitude toward food: Okinawans don't measure food or adhere to rigorous restrictions, and by following the plant-based, 80/20 diet, they are less likely to overeat or struggle with weight control.

Chapter Four

The Okinawa Diet has a few drawbacks.While there are many advantages to a plant-based diet like the Okinawa diet, it's important to be aware of the disadvantages before diving in. Because the meals are low in meat, dairy, and whole grains, certain nutrients like vitamins B and D, calcium, and iron may be lacking. This diet is also high in soy, which may not be ideal for certain populations. (FYI: There is conflicting information on safe levels of soy and its effect on the endocrine system.Before hailing this diet as some sort of wellness panacea, Flowers points out that there's no single reason for Okinawans' good health and long lives—eating habits, exercise routines, relationships, and environment are all possible factors. People in Blue Zones typically take 14,000 to 18,000 steps per day, whereas Americans take about 5,000.Long-term adherence to this diet—specifically, cutting calories to 1,200 calories—would be difficult, if not impossible, to maintain; but, "given the present obesity crisis, most individuals may benefit by dropping some calories from their regular meals." A diet of 1,500 calories may be a better place to begin. In addition, the American diet is more processed and chemically dense than that of other countries. "Learn from the Okinawans and consume more earth-based cuisine."

Chapter Five

Is the Okinawa diet something you should try?

Although the Okinawa diet offers numerous health benefits, some individuals may prefer a diet that is less restricted or low in carbohydrates.The diet's focus on veggies, fiber, and antioxidant-rich foods, as well as its limitations on sugar, processed carbohydrates, and excess fat, may all be beneficial to your health.Okinawan culture promotes regular exercise and mindfulness as well as other lifestyle concepts.It might also have a positive impact on your health.These concepts, however, may be applied to a variety of diverse diets and ways of life.Whether you're not sure if the Okinawa diet is right for you, speak to a nutritionist or healthcare practitioner about developing a plan that's suited to your specific requirements.Can you reduce weight and live longer by following the Okinawa diet?It's no secret that eating more high-fiber foods and fewer processed foods can help you lose weight, but that's not the only reason the Okinawa diet could help you lose weight. Many Okinawans eat according to a Confucian teaching called hara hachi bu, which means eating until you're satisfied rather than full.To prevent overeating, Okinawans do not weigh or measure their food; instead, they opt to eat to live rather than live to eat.Seaweed, bitter melon, shiitake mushrooms, and fatty fish are all high in anti-inflammatory phytochemicals that may help prevent diabetes, heart disease, dementia, and several malignancies.It's also important to note what Okinawans aren't eating. Refined carbs and sugary foods cause blood sugar levels to spike, causing cravings, which leads to a pro-inflammatory state that raises the risk of chronic disease. Limiting red meat also means Okinawans don't consume as much saturated fat, which can lower your risk of heart disease.

Chapter Six

The Okinawa Diet: How to BeginThere's no need to drastically alter your eating habits overnight; instead, consider incorporating more Okinawan foods into your diet; even little adjustments may help your health.Sweet potatoes are a must-have in the kitchen.Replace refined carb sources such as white pasta or white rice with complex carb sources such as buckwheat soba noodles or brown rice on a regular basis.-Vegetables should be a staple in your diet.Most of your meals should include green vegetables such as kale or broccoli, as well as mushrooms. If you want to try out seaweed, try topping your grain bowl with hijiki or adding kombu to your soup.Rethink your protein sources: most of the time, choose for plant-based proteins like tofu, beans, or lentils, with at least a couple portions of fatty fish per week and red meat only on rare occasions.Sugary foods should be avoided.If you're hungry in between meals, try a piece of fruit, a handful of almonds, or a cup of miso soup instead.-

Pour yourself another cup of tea.A basic, unsweetened brew such as jasmine, green, or black tea might help you get a boost of antioxidants.eatablesGrain products and grains• quinoa• rice made of white• noodle soupNoodles made from riceVegetables • seitan – an essential wheat gluten• Sweet potatoes that are purple• Goya/bitter melon (also known as balsam pear)• kombu and mozuku (seaweed)• the root of taro• Hechima/luffa – a cucumber species native to the tropics and subtropics.• Shikwasa (also known as shequasar, flat lemon, or Taiwan tangerine)• okra, a kind of vegetable- • Carrots from Okinawa — long, pale yellow carrots• leeks• tomatillos• Handama is a green and purple leafy vegetable.• Shima rakkyo — a shallot-like root vegetable• leeks• Lettuce• tofu, seasonings, and soy sauce on a plateLegumesLegumes- • soybeans• miso soup• extremely little quantities of soy sauce, since the traditional diet is very low in sodiumFruits- • Bogor pineapple (also known as snack pineapple) - this fruit may be picked apart by hand without the need of a knife.• Shiikwaasaa – commonly known as a flat lemon, this popular citrus fruit contains nobiletin, a flavonoid that has recently been examined in vitro and in animal research for anti-inflammatory and anti-cancer potential.Mangosteens- papaya (fruit)· the fruit of the passionguavas (fruit)• Acerola cherry — high in vitamin C.Meat, fish, and seafood are some of the most popular foods in the world.• fish - gurukun, tuna, and malabar grouper have become famous, yet traditional

Okinawa cookery only employed a little quantity of fish in their dishes (less than a half serving per day)• Meat — a contemporary trend is to consume modest amounts of beef.• goat – an Okinawan delicacyCondiments• koregusu - a distilled liquor containing chili peppers in the bottle; normally, just a few drops are added to dumpling sauce, noodles, and other dishes to offer a touch of flavor.• a tiny bit of soy sauce-
• a teaspoon of sea saltThings to stay away fromMeats:• venison• chickens• items that have been treated• ham with bacon• jamón• prosciutto• hamburgers;• ham• cured meats in generalProducts made with animals:Dairy, such as eggs and•• gouda•• Yogurt Foods that have been processedSugar that has been refinedcereals• cereals for the breakfast• food• cooking oils that have been refinedLegumes:Other foods: • most legumes (excluding soy beans)• the majority of fruits and nuts, as well as seedsMeal plan for an Okinawa diet-MONDAY OF THE WEEKBreakfast• 1/2 cup brown rice boiled; jasmine tea; Basic Miso Soup (wakame potato)Snacking in the middle of the day• Green tea and one low-calorie snack-Lunch• Hijiki brown rice, Shiri-Shiri carrots, and bitter melon, jasmine teaSnack for 3 p.m.• 1 low-calorie snack and a cup of your preferred teaDinner• Spicy Tofu and Summer Veggies; Cucumber and Wakame Vinaigrette, 1/2 cup cooked brown rice, 1/2 papaya; 2 tablespoons low-fat or soy ice cream; jasmine or decaf teaTUESDAYBreakfast• Jasmine tea with soy spinach congeeSnacking in the middle of the day• Green tea

and one low-calorie snackLunch• Sushi roll with jasmine tea from GoyaSnack for 3 p.m.• 1 low-calorie snack teaDinner• Ginkgo-Tofu Supreme or Hawaiian Lemon - Ahi Poke; Nankwa Nbushi; 1/2 cup cooked brown rice; Fuchiba Nantu; jasmine or decaf tea; Nankwa Nbushi; 1/2 cup cooked brown rice; Fuchiba Nantu; jasmine or decaf teaWEDNESDAYBreakfast• 3 oz silken tofu or grilled fish with grated radish; 1/2 cup cooked brown rice; 1 pear; jasmine teaSnacking in the middle of the day• Green tea and 1 low-calorie snackLunch• 1/2 cup cooked brown rice jasmine tea and fragrant Soy-Go Vegetable soup-Snack for 3 p.m.• 1 low-calorie snack; tea of your choiceDinner• Teriyaki Tofu Fingers; Cumin-Chili Cauliflower; 1/2 cup brown rice boiled; 1/8 melon slice; 1/2 cup soy yogurt or low-fat plain yogurt; jasmine or decaf teaTHURSDAYBreakfast1/2 cup brown rice, Mustard Greens Miso Soup, Jasmine TeaSnacking in the middle of the day• Green tea and one low-calorie snack-Lunch• Soba Salad, Miso Soup (wakame Tofu), and Jasmin TeaSnack for 3 p.m.• 1 low-calorie snack teaDinner• Asparagus Tofu Stir-Fry Vegetables; 1/2 cup cooked brown rice; mochi on a leaf; jasmine or decaf teaFRIDAYBreakfast• 1/2 cup brown rice boiled; Okinawa-style gumbo; jasmine teaSnacking in the middle of the day• Green tea and 1 low-calorie snackLunch• 4 pcs. store-bought sushi (no egg sushi) 1 pcs. pear jasmine teaSnack for 3 p.m.• 1 low-calorie snack and a cup of your favorite teaDinner• 1 peach; 2 tbsp low-fat vanilla ice cream or soy ice cream; jasmine or decaf tea; Yuki's Indian Tofu

Curry or Teriyaki Yellowtail with Rice; Asian Okra and Tomato;-SATURDAYBreakfast• 1/2 cup cooked brown rice; jasmine tea; Basic Miso Soup (wakame tofu)Snacking in the middle of the day• Green tea and 1 low-calorie snackLunch• Baby Bok-Choy Stir Fry; 1/2 cup cooked soba noodle; jasmine teaSnack for 3 p.m.• 1 low-calorie snack; tea of your choiceDinner• Wakame Asparagusu; 1/2 cup cooked brown rice; Tapioca Sweet Potato Dessert; jasmine or decaf teaSUNDAYBreakfast• Cantaloupe, jasmine tea, Ogimi Village Sweet Potato Leaf RisottoSnacking in the middle of the day• Green tea and one low-calorie snackLunch• Pita Pizza or Salmon with Nuts and Rice for snacking; jasmine teaSnack for 3 p.m.• 1 low-calorie snack of your choice, with your favorite teaDinner• 1/2 cup cooked brown rice; jasmine or decaf tea; Buddhist Tempe Tofu or Traditional Tsumire Soup; Sweet Amagashi BeansMONDAY IN WEEK TWOBreakfast• 1/2 cup brown rice, jasmine tea, Basic Miso Soup (mustard greens)Snacking in the middle of the day• Green tea and one low-calorie snackLunch• Jasmine tea with baked sweet potatoesSnack for 3 p.m.• 1 low-calorie snack and a cup of your preferred teaDinner• Sloppy Veggie Tofu, Shiitake and Konnyaku Sauté, 1.2 cup cooked brown rice, 1 cup melon cubes sprinkled with 1 teaspoon lime juice, 1/3 cup soy yogurt or low-fat plain yogurt, jasmine or decaf teaTUESDAY-Breakfast• Jasmine tea with soy spinach congeeSnacking in the middle of the day

• Green tea and one low-calorie snackLunch• 1 Vegetarian Noodle Dish with 1/2 cup nodles and plenty of vegetables, plus jasmine teaSnack for 3 p.m.• 1 low-calorie snack and a cup of your preferred teaDinner• Asparagus Tofu Stir-Fry (vegetarian) or Tofu and Peanut Stir-Fry in Oyster Sauce, Cucumber and Wakame Vinaigrette, 1/2 cup cooked brown rice, 1 cup unsweetened fruit salad, jasmine or decaf tea-WEDNESDAYBreakfast• 1 sheet nori laver seaweed cut into eighths, 1/2 cup steamed spinach with 1/2 teaspoon low sodium soy sauce, jasmine teaSnacking in the middle of the day• Green tea and one low-calorie snackLunch• Jasmine tea, fresh tofu spring roll, papaya and shrimp spring rollSnack for 3 p.m.• 1 low-calorie snack and a cup of your preferred teaDinner• Gumbo a la Okinawa Sweet Potato Miso, 1/2 cup cooked brown rice, sweet potato mousse with geren tea sauce, jasmine or decaf teaTHURSDAYBreakfast3 oz. Yuki's Yonaguni Pickles, 1/2 cup cooked brown rice jasmine tea, silken tofu block with green onions minced and 1/2 teaspoon low-sodium soy sauceSnacking in the middle of the day• Green tea and one low-calorie snackLunch• 1 orange jasmine tea, soba salad-Snack for 3 p.m.• 1 low-calorie snack and a cup of your preferred teaDinner• Genmai Tea Shiitake Potato Medley, Asian Okra and Tomato, 1/2 cup cooked brown rice, 1/2 papaya, 2 tablespoons low fat vanilla or soy ice cream, jasmine or decaf teaFRIDAYBreakfast• 1/2 cup cooked brown rice, wakame potato Basic Miso Soup, and jamsine teaSnacking in the middle of the day• Green tea and one low-calorie snack-Lunch• 4 pieces sushi (no egg sushi), 1 apple, and jasmine teaSnack for 3 p.m.• 1 low-calorie snack and a cup of your preferred teaDinner• Sake Shiitake Mushroom Soysteak with 1/2 cup cooked brown rice, Shiri-Shiri Carrot and Bitter Melon, 1 banana halved lengthwise and dusted with 1/2 teaspoon brown sugar, jasmine or decaf teaSATURDAYBreakfast• Miso Soup with 1/2 cooked brown rice, crumbled silken tofu, and spinach, served with jasmine tea.Snacking in the middle of the day• Green tea and one low-calorie snackLunch• 1/2 cup cooked brown rice, jasmine tea, Sweet Potato Miso SoupSnack for 3 p.m.• 1 low-calorie snack and a cup of your preferred tea-Dinner• Goya delight, 1/2 cup cooked brown rice, Darjeeling pudding, jasmine or decaf tea • Fragrant Soy Go Vegetable Soup or Salmon Miso SoupSUNDAYBreakfast• 3 ounces 1/2 cup cooked grilled fish with grated radish or silken tofu with low-sodium soy saucejasmine tea, brown rice, 1 pearSnacking in the middle of the day• 1 cup of green tea (low-cal)Lunch-• Stir-fried sprouts, 1/2 cup brown rice, fresh grapes, and jasmine teaSnack for 3 p.m.• 1 low-calorie snack and a cup of your preferred teaDinner• Tofu from the Buddhist Temple, Wakame Asparagus, Dandelion Spring Rice Mochi on a Leaf, and jasmine or decaf teaRecipes from OkinawaOkinawa Soba (Ski Soba) is a kind of noodle that originated on the island of Okinawa.Time to prepare:2:50Ingredients• 400g egg noodles (0.9 pound) (note 1)• Kamaboko or chikuwa, 120g/5.3oz, sliced to 7mm/14" thick (note 2)8 tablespoons shallots/scallions, finely chopped• Beni shga, 4 tbsp (note 3)Ski (servings for Ski Soba: more than 4)• Pork rib strips weighing 1kg/2.2lb (note 4)• sliced ginger, 30g/1.1ozSki Flavoring is a Japanese term for a flavor that comes from the Japanese• 65ml soy sauce (2.2oz)• 2 tbsp sugar (optional)• mirin, 2 tblsp• 2 tblsp shochuBroth Soba-• 1400 mL broth made from pork that has been boiled• Bonito flakes, 10 g/0.4 oz• 2 tbsp sodium chloride• soy sauce, 2 tbsp• mirin, 2 tblsp• 1 teaspoon sakeInstructions1. Cut the pork rib strip between the rib bones so that each piece has meat on both sides of the bone.2. Fill a pot halfway with water and add the pork pieces.3. Bring to a boil, then reduce to a simmer for 5 minutes.4. Drain the liquid and throw it away.5. Rinse the pork chops thoroughly to remove any scum.6. Clean out the scums from the pot, return the pork to the pot, and stir in the ginger slices.7. Bring water to a boil with enough water to completely cover the pork pieces.8. Reduce to a low heat and cover and cook for 1.5 hours, or until the pork is very tender but not easily broken.9. Take the pork pieces out of the pot and save the broth.Simmered Ski is a type of ski that is made by simulating the movement of1. Place the pork pieces in another large pot or frying pan, preferably large enough to fit them all in without overlapping.2. Bring the ingredients for the Ski Flavouring to a boil in the pot/pan with the pork.3. Lower the heat to low and cook for 5 minutes, turning the pork pieces over to coat them in the flavor.4. Increase the heat to high and cook until the sauce is almost completely gone.5. Remove the heat from the room.SKI BROTH MAKE-UP1. Bring the broth to a boil after adding the bonito flakes.2. Cook for a few minutes on a low heat setting.3. Strain the broth to remove the ginger, bonito flakes, and small pieces of pork.4. Bring the Soba Broth back to a boil with the remaining ingredients.5. Remove the heat from the room.Ski Soba is a Japanese noodles dish.1. In a pot of boiling water, cook the noodles according to the package directions.2. Place noodles in each serving bowl after draining the water.3. Ladle 350ml soba broth into each bowl, then top with simmered ski, kamoaboko/chiku.Okinawan Taco Rice: Quick and Easy15-minute prep time• 170 g minced meat (mixed) or beef mince1 onion, choppedGarlic cloves (two)1 tablespoon Worcestershire sauce (Japanese-style)• 2 tablespoons sweet chilli sauce• Ketchup (two tablespoons)• Sugar, 1 tspLettuce (three leaves)• Tomato (half)• Easy-to-melt cheese (two slices)2 oz.• Nutmeg (approximately 1 teaspoon)-Instructions1. Chop the onion and garlic into small pieces.2. In a frying pan, heat some vegetable oil and cook until the chicken is done.3. Add the minced meat and cook until it is golden brown.4. Combine the ingredients and sprinkle with nutmeg.5. Combine everything in a bowl.6. Arrange a slice of cheese on top of the cooked rice without cutting it.7. Melt the cheese in the microwave on high for 30 seconds.8. Place the mixture from Step 2 on top of the melted cheese.9. Toss on shredded lettuce, diced tomatoes, and a fried egg.10. Toss with ketchup and season with salt and pepper.Rice with Tofu and Vegetables17 minutes for preparationIngredients• Tofu (firm): 150 gKidney beans (30 g)• Onion (50g)• Tomato (half)-Garlic clove, 1/2• 1 tsp. salt, plus 1 tsp. pepper• 2 teaspoon chili powder• 1 tbsp Worcestershire sauce (Japanese style)• Ketchup, 1 tbsp• Soy sauce, 1 tsp• Vegetable oil (1/2 tsp)1 brown rice bowlAvocado, cut into five slices• Cherry tomatoes and lettuce (two leaves each)• Shredded cheese, 1 bunch-Instructions1. Microwave the tofu for 2 minutes at 600 W after wrapping it in two layers of paper towels.2. Remove the paper towels and replace them.3. Chop the onions, tomatoes, and garlic until they are finely chopped.4. In a frying pan, heat the oil and cook the garlic, onions, tofu, and tomatoes until the liquid has evaporated.5. Combine the kidney beans with the rest of the ingredients.6. Toss in the above-mentioned ingredients, then add the soy sauce after the flavors have been evenly distributed.7. Pile the rice on the plate, then add Step 4 to the top.8. Combine the avocado, tomatoes, cheese, and lettuce in a large mixing bowl.Taco Rice with Vegetables-30 minutes of preparationIngredients• Koya tofu (one block)-1 Carrot, small1 onion, chopped1 green pepper, chopped-Lettuce (three leaves)• 1 leaf of the baby• 5 tomatoes, cherry• Avocado (half)• Cilantro (quarter-bunch)• 1 tablespoon of extra virgin olive oil• 50 milliliters (milliliters) water• Ketchup (three tablespoons)• 2 tablespoons Worcestershire sauce (Japanese style)• 1 tbsp. chili powder• Soy sauce, 2 tsp• 1 teaspoon of salt and freshly ground black pepperWarm brown rice, 2 servings1 tbsp. mayonnaise (soy)• Cheese (one)• Tortilla chips (1 Tortilla)Instructions1. Soak the koya tofu in warm water for at least 30 minutes.2. Before cutting, wash and drain the vegetables thoroughly.3. Half the cherry tomatoes and cut the lettuce into thick strips.4. Avocados have a tendency to turn brown when cut, so save it for later.5. [Vegetarian Taco Meat] Drain the tofu and puree it in a food processor.6. Chop the vegetables with the arrows finely.7. Heat some olive oil in a frying pan.8. Stir-fry the finely chopped vegetables marked, then add the blended tofu and stir-fry everything together.-9. Once the meat is cooked, add the seasoning ingredients marked with and continue to stir fry while bringing to a boil.10. Adjust the seasoning with a pinch of salt and pepper as needed to keep the meat tasting good.11. Finally, cut the avocado; if you have any, a few drops of lemon juice will help keep it from turning brown.12. Don't overdo it with the avocado, or it will become too sour.13. Place the brown rice on a plate once it has been cooked.14. Place the vegetables marked with an asterisk on top, followed by the taco "meat" and finally the soy mayonnaise.Finish with tortilla chips as a finishing touch.For taco rice or tacos, use taco meat.15 minutes for preparation-Ingredients• 350 g beef mince1 onion, choppedGarlic cloves (two)• 2 tablespoons Worcestershire sauce (Japanese style)-• Ketchup (two tablespoons)• 1 tablespoon of Sake• Chili powder (1 tbsp)• Soy sauce, 1 tsp1 teaspoon curry powder• 1 teaspoon of salt and freshly ground black pepper• 1 tblsp. olive oilInstructions1. Chop the onion and garlic into small pieces.2. In a frying pan, heat the vegetable oil and slowly sauté the garlic.3. Stir in the meat and onion once the garlic has become fragrant.4. Season with salt and pepper, then stir-fry until the clumps are broken up.5. Combine the ingredients once the meat has begun to change color.6. Adjust the flavor with additional salt and pepper if necessary.Tacos with fajitas y pollo asado, risotto10 minutes to prepareIngredients5 tortillas de mazFajitas (two)• 1 breast de poulet3/4 onion, diced• Green bell pepper, 1/2 cup• Pepper and lemon• Cilantro and raw onionsa lime (half)Instructions1. Begin with half-cooked fajitas, then add the chicken breast while both the chicken and the fajitas are cooking, followed by the onion and lemon pepper seasoning.2. When it's done, put it in your corn tortillas and top it with cilantro, raw onion, or whatever else you like. You can also top it with whatever salsa you want.Goya sautéed (Goya Chanpuru)15 minutes for preparationIngredients• 1/2 goya (20 cm) (cut lengthwise in half, remove seeds, cut into 35mm slices)• Tofu (firm) (200 g)• Beef or ham, 100–150 g• 1/2 onion, cut in half• Carrot, 1/4• 12 egg yolks, whisked-Seasonings:• 1 tablespoon of sake• Soy sauce, 1 tbsp• Oyster sauce, 1/21 tbsp• 1 tablespoon vegetable or olive oil for tofu frying• sesame oil, 1 tblsp• bonito flakes (dried) to use as a garnish• seasonings (salt, pepper)Instructions1. Rub salt into the goya, then set aside for 10 minutes.2. Rinse and drain thoroughly.3. In a skillet over medium heat, heat the oil (vegetable or olive oil) and stir fry the tofu until golden brown.-4. Remove and set aside the tofu from the pan.5. In the same pan, heat the sesame oil, then add the beef, onion, carrot, and goya and cook for 12 minutes, stirring occasionally.6. Return the tofu to the pan, then stir in the seasonings.7. Pour in the beaten egg and quickly stir to combine.Salt & pepper to taste.9. Top with bonito flakes that have been dried.Taco Rice Casserole is a dish that combines the flavors of tacos and1 hour 15 minutes preparation timeIngredients• Ground Beef, 2 lb.1 chopped onion• 1 Zucchini Shredded• 2 C Corn• 1 Can Black beans (drained) (drained)• 1 Can Rotel• 1 Package Taco seasoning• Sodium• 4 C Cooked rice• Handfuls shredded cheese• 2 9x13 pansInstructions1. Brown beef. Add in Onion and zucchini and cook until soft.2. Stir in taco seasoning.3. Add corn, tomatoes and beans.4. Spray 2 pans, spoon 2 C rice into the bottom of each pan.5. Spoon the meat mixture over the rice.6. Top with shredded cheese.7. If you want to eat right away: bake covered at 350 for 25 min.8. If freeze: let thaw overnight in fridge.9. Bake at 350 for 45 min covered.10. Then remove foil and cook until top is nice and brown.DOUGHNUTS OF OKINAWAN40 minutes of preparationINGREDIENTS• oil (for deep frying) (for deep frying)• 4 eggs• ¾ cup milk• ¾ teaspoon vanilla• 4cups flour• 2 cups sugar• 3 ½ tablespoons baking powder• ¼ teaspoon saltInstructions• In a deep fryer or deep skillet, heat oil to 350 F or until hot.• In a large bowl, beat eggs, milk, and vanilla. Sift flour, sugar, baking powder and salt.• Add to egg mixture; stir until dry ingredients are moistened and dough is smooth.• Drop teaspoonfuls of dough into the hot oil; fry until golden brown and doughnuts rise to the surface.• Drain on paper towel lined plates and serve hot, but they are also good cooled down, you can buy them either way there on Okinawa!Sweet potatoes from Okinawa1 hour of preparationIngredients• 4 pounds Okinawa (purple) sweet potatoes or white sweet potatoes, scrubbed• 2 limes• 1/4 cup butter• Hawaiian red clay salt or sea saltInstructions1. Bring a large pot of water to a boil over high heat.2. Prick sweet potatoes with a fork and boil until tender when pierced, 30 to 35 minutes.3. Drain.4. While potatoes are boiling, grate zest from limes and set aside; then squeeze juice from limes and set aside.5. When potatoes are cool enough to handle, peel and slice into 1/2-in.-thick slices.6. Arrange on a platter, cover with foil, and put in a 200° oven to keep warm.7. Melt butter in a small saucepan over medium heat until foaming. Stir in zest and cook until fragrant, 1 minute.8. Remove from heat and stir in lime juice.9. Drizzle lime butter over potatoes and sprinkle with salt.Shortbread from Okinawa with salt45 minutes for preparationIngredients• 80 glard or vegetable shortening• 60 gsoft dark brown sugar• 150 gplain flour• 1 tspsea salt flakesInstructions1. Heat your oven to 160°C.2. In a medium saucepan, heat the lard and brown sugar together over low heat until liquid and combined.3. Add the flour and mix to a soft dough.4. Roll the dough between two sheets of baking paper to around 1cm thick and cut into 8cm x 3cm batons (using a crinkle cutter if possible) (using a crinkle cutter if possible).5. Transfer the biscuits to a baking sheet and scatter with sea salt, lightly pressing it into the top of the biscuit.6. Bake for around 25 minutes until firm.7. Allow to cool before serving.Pork & Vegetables Champroo (Chanpurū) Preparation time25 minutesIngredients• 1 tablespoon Oil• 1 block (450 g) Firm Tofu• 200 g beef thinly sliced• Salt & Black Pepper• 1 Onion• 1/2 Carrot

• 2 Cabbage Leaves OR other Vegetables, such as Garlic chives, spring onion, okra, and other vegetables• Katsuobushi (Bonito) Dashi Powder (1/2 teaspoon)• 2 tablespoons soy sauce (adjust the quantity to your preference)• 3 egg yolks, whiskedInstructions1.Vegetables should be cut into tiny strips or bite-size chunks.2.Firm Tofu should be cut or broken into bite-size pieces.3.Season thinly sliced beef with salt and pepper before cutting into bite-size pieces. In a small mixing dish, lightly whisk the eggs.4.Dashi Powder and Soy Sauce should be ready to use.5.Is everything in order? You may now begin cooking. Cook Tofu pieces till brown in a wok or big frying pan over medium high heat, season with salt, and transfer to a platter.6.In a frying pan, brown the meat.7.When the steak is done, toss in the vegetables and stir-fry. Return the Tofu when the vegetables are soft.8.Stir in the Dashi Powder and Soy Sauce, then pour in the whisked Eggs.9.Allow it to sit for a few minutes without stirring until the Egg is almost set, then whisk to mix.Rice in Tacos15 minutes for preparationIngredients• Beef Mince (500 g) OR Beef & Beef Mince (500 g)• 1 tablespoon of canola oil• a single onion• 1 garlic clove, coarsely chopped• 2 tablespoons tomato paste• 4 portions of freshly cooked rice• 2-3 chopped lettuce leaves• 2 tomatoes, peeled and chopped into tiny pieces• 1 avocado, peeled and chopped into tiny pieces• Cheddar cheese that has been shreddedSalsa de Tacos• 2 tablespoons cumin powder• 2 tablespoons coriander powder• 1 teaspoon garlic powder• a teaspoon of paprika• Cayenne Pepper (optional): 1/8 teaspoon• 1 teaspoon kosher saltInstructions1.In a large frying pan, heat the oil over medium-high heat and saute the onion and garlic for a few minutes before adding the beef mince and cooking until the beef changes color.2.Stir in the spice mixture and Tomato Paste for a few minutes.-3.Place the Freshly Cooked Rice on a platter, then top with the Beef combination, lettuce, tomato, avocado, and shredded cheese.4.Enjoy with Taco Salsa drizzled on top.Goya Chanpuru is a fictional character created by Goya Chanpuru20 minutes for preparation3 servings of ingredients1 goya is required• 2 beaten eggs• 300 g pork chops, cut• Bonito flakes (about a handful)• 200 grams of tofu• sesame seeds and oil• pepper and salt• a little soy sauceInstructions1.Cut the pork into 4cm slices, the goya into 1cm slices, and the tofu into bite-size pieces.2.1 tsp sesame oil for stir-frying the meat3.When the meat is done, add the tofu and goya to the pan and simmer for 3 minutes together.4.Season the tofu with salt and pepper when it starts to acquire a bit charcoal.5.Pour the beaten egg and bonito flakes into the pan, then evenly pour the soy sauce from the pan's edge.Tacos of carne and arroz con arroz y arroz y arTime to prepare: 2 hoursIngredients• 3 cups white rice• 2 onion slices• 4 garlic cloves• 8 tblspn of olive oil• 4 servings of maggi• Add a pinch of salt• Herbs and spices• 2 c. tomatoes + 1 tsp. pepper pasteTo prepare the meat• 3 beef ribs of varying sizes• 4 pcs garlic cloves• 2 onion slices• 1 scotch bonnet pepper• 1 pound of maggi• 1 tablespoon curry powder• 1/2 teaspoon cinnamon• 1/2 gallon of water• Add a pinch of saltDressing made with mayonnaise• 4 tablespoons mayonnaise• 3 garlic cloves• 1 tablespoon red chilli flakes• 1 scotch bonnet pepper• a half teaspoon of black pepper• 1/2 teaspoon of pepper paste• Add a pinch of saltWraps made with tortillas (tacos)• 1 cup of flour• 1/2 teaspoon of baking powder• 3 tblpsn olive oil• Add a pinch of salt• Drinking water-For the beef, follow these instructions:1.In a saucepan, pour in the oil.2.Add the onions and garlic and cook for a minute.3.Stir in the meat and seasonings for 2 to 3 minutes.4.Mix in the Scotch bonnet.5.Cook till soft by adding water and covering it.For the rice, follow these instructions:1.In a saucepan, heat the oil, then add the rice and stir until golden brown. Drain in a strainer.2.Add all of the rice ingredients and simmer for 2 minutes, then add the rice and enough water to cover the top of the rice.3.Cook until the vegetables are tender.To make the tortilla, combine the following ingredients.1.Combine all of the ingredients in a large mixing bowl.2.Add a little water at a time until a soft dough forms.3.10 minutes of kneading the dough4.Allow it to rest for 5 minutes before serving.5.Roll it out and bake it in a pan for 112 minutes on each side.-

To make the mayonnaise, combine the following ingredients in a mixing bowl.1. Mix all of the ingredients together.The tacos arrangement is as follows:1.Toss with the mayonnaise dressing.2.The meat comes next, followed by the rice. The top of the wrap should be egg washed.3.Butter your skillet, put the tacos, and bake over low heat until golden brown, then serve.Rice for Tacos35 minutes of preparationIngredients-

• Rice paper (six sheets) (for summer rolls)• Cooked rice (prepared with 2 cups rice)• 150 g lean ground beef• a single avocado• 6 pieces miniature tomato• chips from tacos (tortilla chips)• mozzarella cheese for pizzaseasonings• 1/2 tea spoon granule type chicken bouillon• ketchup (three table spoons)• a half teaspoon of cuminInstructions1.In a Teflon pan, roast ground beef and drain any extra fat.2.Season the ground beef with a variety of spices.3.Prepare the rice.4.Cut the avocado into slices.5.Half-cut the cherry tomatoes.6.Tortilla chips are a great snack.7.Soften the skin of the summer rolls (rice paper) and form a long bale of rice.8.Make a hole in the center of the rice and fill it with ground meat.9.Place the pizza cheese on top.10.Finally, add taco chips to the mix (tortilla chips),11.Place the avocado on the rice's top edge.12.Place a small tomato on top.13.Everything should be wrapped in summer rolls. It will not collapse if you wrap it tightly. You may also use dry curry.Carrots from Okinawa Preparation time: 15 minutes-INGREDIENTS• 3 carrots, medium to large in size• 1 egg, lightly whisked• 1 tablespoon soy sauce• sesame oil, 1 tsp• 1 5 oz tuna in oil canned tuna – you'll only use about 1/2 of it; save the rest for snacking!• a pinch of salt• a sprinkle of black pepper• water for the carrots to be cooked• 1 sliced green onion to serve as a garnishINSTRUCTIONS1.Carrots should be peeled and julienned. The finer you julienne your carrots, the faster they'll cook!2.In a small bowl, whisk one egg and set it aside.3.Preheat a skillet to medium-high heat.4.Fill the skillet with the oil from the tuna can and heat it up.5.Once the oil is hot, toss in the carrots.6.Stir fry for about 10 minutes, or until the vegetables are softened.7.To help the carrots cook, drizzle in a little water here and there. You don't want it to be watery, so if you add water, make sure it burns off.8.When the carrots are soft and pliable, add the tuna and stir to break it up.9.Add the soy sauce, sesame oil, and a pinch of salt and pepper after that.10.Finally, pour in your whisked egg and continue to stir until it is fully cooked.11.Remove from the oven and serve immediately with a green onion garnish!-Tofu and Veggies from Okinawa15 minutes for preparation-Ingredients• 1 cup carrots, peeled and sliced• 2 cups thinly sliced white or yellow onion• 1 12-14 oz package firm tofu in water, drained and cut into 1/2 inch cubes• 1-2 tablespoons extra virgin olive oil• 1 tablespoon butter is optional, but adds flavor to the dish.• salt and freshly ground black pepper• Soy sauce, 2 tbsp.• 1-2 bunches green onions, white and green sections, chopped diagonally into 1″ pieces• Optional garnish: sesame seedsInstructions1.By cleaning, slicing, and putting away all of the veggies and tofu.2.Preheat a medium to large sauté or fry pan to medium-high heat.3.In a separate pan, melt the butter and add the olive oil.4.Melt the butter in a small saucepan over low heat.5.Carrots and sliced yellow or white onion should be carefully added to the pan.6.Stir-fry for 3-4 minutes, until veggies begin to soften, seasoning with salt and pepper.7.Set aside the vegetables from the pan.-8.Toss the tofu once or twice in the pan while cooking for 3-4 minutes total.9.Return to pan heat for another minute, without tossing, or the tofu will break apart.10.Heat should be turned off.11.Serve immediately with gohan (rice) and additional sides if preferred, along with chopped green onions and sesame seeds (optional).Chanpuru with Fish Sauce and Asian Somen Noodles20 minutes for preparationIngredients-• 1 Somen noodle bundle• 60 g pork belly or beef offcuts-• Komatsuna (two bundles)• Vegetable oil (1 tbsp)1 minced garlic clove• 1 tbsp. ginger, mincedTakanotsume (half) (sliced)• 1 1/2 tsp. fish sauce• 1 tblsp. vinaigrette• Shaoxing wine (about 2/3 tsp)• 1/2 tsp sodium chloride• 1/2 teaspoon stock powder (chicken soup)• 1 cayenne• 1 lemon, squeezedInstructions-

1.Combine all of the spices in a bowl and mix well.2.Beef should be cut into appropriate portions.3.Cook the somen noodles for one minute less than the box suggests.4.Drain well after rinsing with cold water.5.In a skillet, heat the vegetable oil and cook the minced garlic, ginger, and sliced red chile pepper, being careful not to burn them.6.Stir in the meat after it has become fragrant.7.Add the somen noodles after the meat has started to brown.8.Add the chopped komatsuna to the pan with the seasoning from Step 1, and season with pepper.9.It's done if you toss quickly.Taco Rice Is Good For You30 minutes of preparationMeat sauce ingredients200 g beef mince• 1 sliced onion (big)• 1/2 bamboo stalk, sliced and blanched1 tin With your little hands, smush the tomatoes together. Tomatoes in can1 garlic clove• 1 Any herbs and spices you happen to have on hand1 bay leaf is needed• 1 tblsp. wine or saké• 1 tsp. ketchup, Japanese Worcestershire sauce, soy sauce, sugar, salt, and pepperSalsaTomatoes, 1 cup (to taste)• 1 onion, finely chopped and placed in a basin of water (to taste)• 1 olive oil swish• 1 tsp. lemon juice, with a sprig of parsley (optional)• 1 tsp. salt, 1 tsp. pepper1 tbsp. TabascoChoose your own vegetables• 1 (to taste). julienne is a term used to describe a cut that is about j Celery, lettuce-Toppings• 1 tbsp. pizza or cheese (to taste)Instructions1.Let's begin by preparing the pork sauce.2.Without using any oil, stir-fry the ground beef.3.Any rendered fat must be drained.-4.Stir in the onion, bamboo shoot, and a splash of sake after seasoning with salt and finely powdered black pepper.5.Add as much as you wish of whichever herbs and spices you have on hand.6.Red chili powder, oregano, paprika, nutmeg, and black pepper are all good additions, but the chili powder is required.7.Add one bay leaf and one can of crushed tomatoes (juice included).8.Ketchup, Worcestershire sauce, soy sauce, sugar, salt, and pepper are all used to flavor the dish. Taste and adjust the amount to your liking.9.Just taste it while it cooks, even if you didn't measure the ingredients. It's done when the pan has no more liquid in it.10.Make the salsa by combining the ingredients.11.Combine the ingredients for the salsa, season to taste with salt and pepper, and serve.12.Toss in a pinch of Tabasco, then season with salt and pepper to taste.13.In a bowl, combine rice, salsa, a substantial quantity of the meat sauce, cheese, and parsley.14.Finished!! To taste, add a little extra Tabasco.Miso Is The Key In This Healthy Chanpuru Tofu Stir-FryTime to prepare:Ingredients• Firm tofu, half a block (150 g)• Kiriboshi daikon (dry shredded daikon radish) (25 grams)• Chinese garlic chives (half a bunch)Carrot (30 g)2 mushrooms (shitake)• 1 tablespoon Miso• 1 tablespoon of Sake• Mirin, 2 tbsp• 2 tablespoons dashi stock (Japanese)- • 1 teaspoon ginger juice• Sesame oil, 1 tblsp• 1–2 tbsp sesame seeds, groundInstructions1.Microwave for 1 minute after wrapping the tofu in paper towels. Allow to cool before continuing.2.To rehydrate the dried kiriboshi daikon radish, soak it in water for a few minutes before cutting it into bite-size pieces.3.Combine all of the specified ingredients in a bowl.-4.Cut the Chinese chives into 1cm lengths at the base and 3cm lengths at the leafy section.5.Thinly slice the carrots into rectangles.6.Shitake mushrooms should be finely sliced.7.In a frying pan, heat the sesame oil and add the carrots and daikon radish.8.On a medium to high heat, stir cook the ingredients.-9.Continue stirring frying with the bottom portion of the Chinese chives.10.Stir in the leaves Chinese chives.11.Toss in the tofu, breaking it up with your hands.12.To avoid breaking up the tofu chunks, gently stir.13.Remove from the fire and stir in the ingredients listed.14.Transfer to a serving plate and finish with the sesame seeds.On Toast, Taco RiceTime to prepare:Ingredients• 1 pound shredded cheese (pizza style)• 1 tomato, diced (1 cm)• 1 pound ground beef with ketchup tasteInstructions1.Toast the ingredients on a slice of bread!-2.After cooking taco rice for my lunchbox, I prepared this with what was left over.3.On top of the bread, you may use as much as you like!Taco Rice for a Trendy Lunch12 minutes for preparationIngredients• 100 g beef mince1 onion, chopped1 tsp. garlic chips• 1 tsp. salt, plus 1 tsp. pepper• Lettuce (quarter of a head)1 tomato, peeled• Easy-to-melt cheese (two slices)• 2 fresh eggs (hot)• Sweet chili sauce, 2 tbsp• Ketchup, 1 tbsp• Soy sauce, 1 tbspInstructions1.Sauté the garlic chips in vegetable oil in a frying pan.2.Stir-fry the meat and onions together.3.-Using a paper towel, mop up any extra oil after the chicken is fully cooked.4.In a mixing bowl, combine all of the ingredients.-

5.Layer the rice, pork, and cheese slices on top of each other on plates. Microwave for approximately 30 seconds at 550 W until the cheese melts.6.Add the lettuce and tomatoes to the dish, shredding the lettuce and chopping the tomatoes into 1-centimeter bits. Serve immediately with a fried egg on top.7.If desired, serve with a dash of Tabasco sauce.-Rice bowls stuffed with fish tacos30 minutes of preparation-Ingredients1 cup brown rice (uncooked)• 1 3/4 cup of liquid• 1 pound Skin taken from mahi mahi• chipotle chile powder (about 1/4 teaspoon)• Garlic powder (1 teaspoon)• 1 tsp. paprika (smoked)• 1/2 teaspoon sodium chloride• 1 teaspoon black pepper, freshly ground• Canola oil, 1 tbsp.• mashed avocado (two avocados)• lime juice, 2 tbsp.• 2 cups thinly chopped purple cabbage• 1 cup jicama, thinly sliced1 roma tomato, diced• Onions, freshly pickedDressing: Cilantro Lime• 1 red onion, chopped1 garlic clove is required1 cup cilantro, chopped• Canola oil (about 1/4 cup)• 2 tbsp lime juice (fresh)-• red wine vinegar, 2 tblsp.1 tsp honey• 2 tblsp. mustard (dijon)1 tsp. salt• a sprinkle of cumin powderInstructions1.Fill a microwave-safe bowl halfway with water and rice.2.Microwave for 10 minutes on HIGH power.3.Allow it cool for a few minutes before fluffing.4.12 teaspoon salt, 14 teaspoon black pepper, chipotle chile powder, garlic powder, smoked paprika, 12 teaspoon salt5.To mix ingredients, whisk them together.6.Dry the fish well before applying the spice mixture to both sides.7.-Preheat a medium-large skillet over high heat.8.1 tablespoon canola oil, then insert cooked fish in pan gently.9.For 4-5 minutes on each sides, sear.10.Allow to cool in the pan.11.-14 cup canola oil, lime juice, red wine vinegar, honey, dijon mustard, 14 teaspoon salt, and cumin in a food processor12.-Until smooth, blend. Remove the item from circulation.13.2 tablespoons lime juice, mashed avocado14.Toss with a pinch of salt and pepper, to taste.15.Combine all ingredients and mix well.16.Fill the bowls with 12 cup rice, one filet of fish, a big scoop of avocado mash, and a pinch of salt and pepper.14 cup sliced jicama, 12 cup purple cabbage, 14 cup diced tomato17.-Serve with a drizzle of dressing.

CPSIA information can be obtained
at www.ICGtesting.com
Printed in the USA
LVHW060741060422
715401LV00015B/569

9 781804 384596